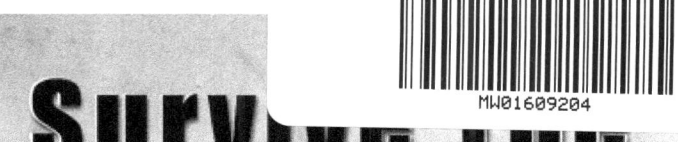

Survive The Coming Storm

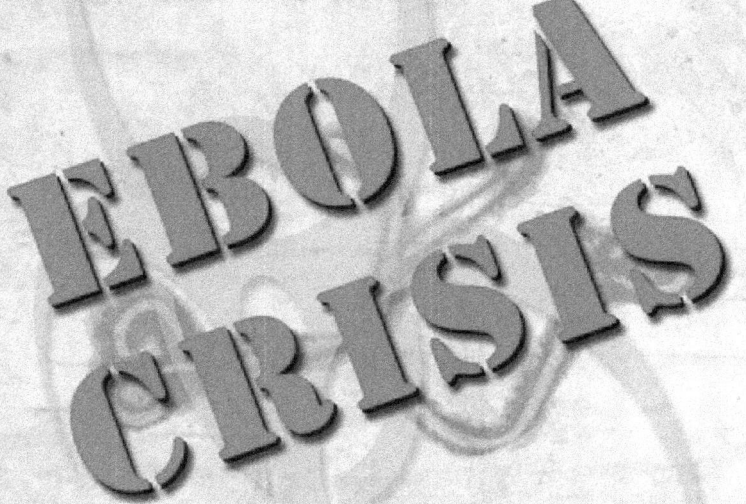

EBOLA CRISIS

Preparing Now...
Before It Is To Late

By Ray Gano

Forward By Michael Snyder

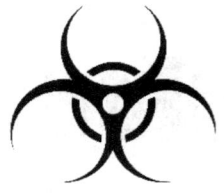

Survive The Coming Storm - EBOLA CRISIS

A Prepper's Guide on How To Prepare For
A Killer Global Pandemic and Treat At Home

By Ray Gano

Foreword By Michael Snyder

Survive The Coming Storm - EBOLA CRISIS

A Prepper's Guide on How To Prepare For A Killer Global Pandemic and Treat At Home

©2014 by Ray Gano

Cover Designed by Ray Gano

All Scripture used in this book is taken from The Authorized King James Bible

Medical Disclaimer

Please note that all information in this report / eBook is for educational purposes only. This content is intended to supplement, not to replace, consultation with a physician. You should not use information in this report / eBook to diagnose or treat a health problem or disease. We encourage you to consult your health care provider with any questions or concerns you may have regarding your condition. The information contained in this report / eBook is not intended to cover all possible uses, directions, precautions, warnings, drug interactions, allergic reactions, or adverse effects.

=-=-=-=-=-=-=-=-=-=-=

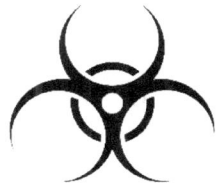

"When it happens you will know that it is true, by then it will be too late."

An Old Russian Proverb

But if any provide not for his own, and specially for those of his own house,

he hath denied the faith, and is worse than an infidel.

1 Timothy 5:8

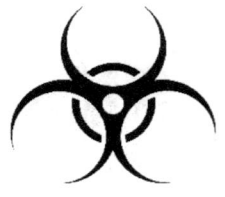

Dedication

First and foremost I dedicate this to my Lord and Savior, Jesus Christ. He paid the ultimate price by shedding His blood and dying for us.
It is our reasonable service that we live our lives completely for Him.

Secondly, I dedicate this book to my wife who puts up with some of my hair brained ideas and also, my God inspired profound truths. Thank you for standing by my side all these years. They have been wonderful and cannot imagine being with anyone other than you.

To my kids and grandkids, we love you and know that you have it in you to survive the coming storms. We raised you with the knowledge.

To my Prophezine readers and PZ Insiders, thank you for being there, for keeping us in prayer and supporting us through all of the ups and downs that a ministry experiences. Many of you have become good friends and I look forward growing more friendships.

To you the reader, I hope that what I share in this book will provide nuggets of truth that will help you to "Survive The Coming Storm."

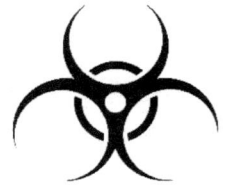

Table of Contents

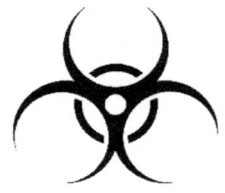

Endorsements

Ray's new guide for preparing for this next storm is not only timely but well thought out.

Taking after the sound advice of his previous book, "Survive The Coming Storm – A Value of A Preparedness Lifestyle" he helps you separate fact from fiction and in a logical format.

This book will help you to think through what you need to have available to prepare you and your family for a pandemic; whatever the cause of it is.

The information is this book is relevant for everyone; whether you are single, in charge of a large family or a medical provider.

After practicing for 25 years as a Physician Assistant, I have also realized that the patients who take responsibility for their health and have a better mental attitude towards whatever they are dealing with, fare much better overall- no matter what the situation is. Ray gives you the information you need to be mentally and physically as ready as possible.

Deborah Hunter PA-C

The word 'Ebola' brings to mind suffering and death in far off places that don't affect most modern nations, cities, or families. The truth is that today there are no far off places. Travelers go from one corner of the globe to the opposite corner in less than 24 hours. That means dreadful disease can touch anywhere at any time. The key to dealing with the threat of Ebola is to be as prepared as possible, not to waste time worrying, and to trust God with the outcome.

Reading 'Ebola Crisis' by Ray Gano will provide you with a good foundation for setting up a plan to manage an Ebola crisis or any pandemic should you ever need to.

When Ray writes a book he can be trusted to fully research the subject and present the material in a manner that is truthful and understandable. 'Ebola Crisis' definitely provides honest helpful information. Whether you are a seasoned prepper or someone just realizing that a global pandemic is a definite possibility you will find the book to be an excellent resource.

Barbara Henderson – Author & Journalist

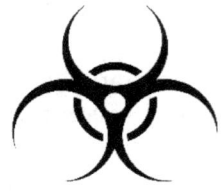

Forward by Michael Snyder

The Economic Collapse

There have been lots of health scares in the past. One that comes to mind is the swine flu hysteria that we witnessed just a few years ago. But something seems very different about this crisis. The truth is that if you get Ebola, you are probably going to die. Health officials tell us that the death rate for Ebola can be up to 90 percent, and so far during this current crisis it is over 50 percent. At the moment, there is no publicly available vaccine and no cure for Ebola. It is a vicious killing machine that is both silent and brutally efficient.

And according to the experts you can be carrying it around for up to three weeks before you even know that you have the disease. In fact, Ebola victims can be walking around and acting normally up to just a short time before their deaths. The person sitting next to you on a plane or walking past you in the grocery store could have Ebola without showing any visible symptoms.

Needless to say, this is pretty much an ideal disease for causing fear. If this virus starts spreading inside the United States, it is going to cause a wave of panic unlike anything else we have seen in post-World War II history. Schools will be shut down, nearly all public gatherings will be cancelled and nearly everyone will want to stay home as much as possible.

If the panic lasted for a number of months (or years) it would have the potential to absolutely crash our economy. Shopping malls and supermarkets would be virtually empty due to fear. Many people would not even want to leave their homes to go to their jobs because of the risk of catching a virus which could easily kill them.

And of course our financial markets would crash in such an environment and we would experience the worst credit crunch that we have ever seen. Just think about it. Nobody would want to lend money to anyone in the midst of a raging Ebola pandemic.

But just about every major transaction in our economy depends on the flow of credit. Without the ability to go into debt, most of us would not be able to buy a home, buy a vehicle or go to college.

And if the federal government implemented strict travel restrictions to combat the spread of the virus, that could result in empty store shelves very rapidly – especially in rural areas. Most people don't realize how extremely dependent we are on the trucking industry to bring us the things that we need. If that system broke down, a large segment of the population would be in deep trouble. Many families out there could only last a few weeks (or even a few days) on the food that they have in their homes right now.

I hope that you will listen to what Ray has to say in this book. There are way too many people out there that are apathetic at the moment. A few years ago, it was quite trendy to be a "prepper" and lots of people were jumping on board. But over the past couple of years sales of emergency food and supplies are way down across the industry. It seems like most Americans have pretty much forgotten about the financial crisis of 2008 and just assume that whatever problems that we had back then have been fixed. And way too many people have blind faith in our government officials.

A lot of people that I hear from are convinced that the U.S. government can handle pretty much whatever comes our way and that because of our advanced technology that we don't have anything to worry about.

But just because things have always been a certain way does not mean that they will always be that way.

There is something called "normalcy bias" that those of us that are trying to warn America about what is coming are constantly battling. Most people underestimate the potential for disaster because they have never experienced one. Therefore, they do not prepare adequately. For as long as most of us can remember, things have been really good in this country. There have been "scares" in the past, but most of them have never really panned out. And the ones that did turn out to be something passed after a while.

So many people are openly wondering why they should be alarmed this time. In fact, even in the "prepper community" many are dismissing this Ebola threat as just a bunch of "hype".

And I would love it if that does indeed turn out to be the case. I don't want to see an Ebola pandemic in America. I don't want to see mass panic and mass fear. I don't want to see millions of people die. I don't want to see families torn apart and our economy destroyed by this virus.

But the reality of the matter is that we would be quite foolish not to take this threat seriously. As I write this, the number of confirmed Ebola cases and the number of confirmed Ebola deaths is growing at an exponential rate. Let us pray that they find a way to contain this disease, because if not it could very easily turn into a global nightmare. We could literally be facing the greatest health crisis that any of us have ever seen in our entire lifetimes.

On a personal note, this summer my wife and I felt much more of an urgency to store up emergency food and supplies than we ever have before. Of course we have always been prepping, but this summer we have put our efforts into overdrive. Now with a potential Ebola crisis on the horizon, we are very thankful for how hard we have been working.

If an Ebola outbreak starts sweeping across America, you need to be prepared to stay at home as much as possible for an extended period of time. You are going to need lots of food and supplies. And you will want to stock up on anything that you may need to combat the disease while suppliers still have them.

I am thankful that Ray has decided to write this book. I think that it is very timely and that you are going to get a lot out of it.

Once again, let us hope and pray that this crisis fizzles out at some point.

But what if it doesn't?

There is hope in understanding what is happening and there is hope in getting prepared.

Get prepared while you still can, because time is running out.

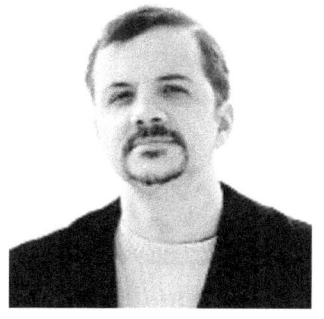

Michael Snyder

The Economic Collapse
http://theeconomiccollapseblog.com/

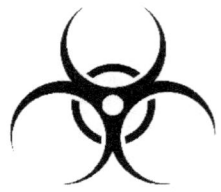

A Few Words From The Author About This Book

My name is Ray Gano; I am a prepper and have been a prepper pretty much all my life. My mother was raised during the great depression because of that was always a frugal person. She would can up and dehydrate food, setting it aside for "a rainy day."

One of my most vivid memories growing up was during the economic recession we had in the mid-1960s. Life for us was pretty hard. I remember us going behind grocery stores and picking out old fruit and vegetables. We would pick mustard greens, black berries, crab apples, anything that was growing on the side of the road we would stop and pick it. There was a butcher in town that used to save beef bones for us and my mom would gather us around the stove and make "nail soup."

Nail soup was a big deal back then. We all helped clean up the old vegetables, cut away bad pieces and keep the good parts. Mom would then have us carefully put the veggies we cut up into the pot. Finally she would pick one of us kids to take the magic nail from the window sill and put it in the pot. See, the nail was magic and that is what made the "Nail Soup" taste so good.

The real ingredient was the best of all; it was my mother's love.

Another point when I was growing up was when my father contracted Hong Kong Flu. This was around the same time in the mid to late 1960's. I remember my mom quarantining the room and keeping us kids away. Only she could go into the room and she worked hard to keep the house sterile and germ free.

Many people died from the Hong Kong Flu, which come to find out was a strain of H1N1 Spanish Flu. The same H1N1 that we still have today that many believe will eventually mutate again into a more harmful form of H1N1.

Over the years I was drawn to home remedies, and back woods cures. I started to learn about all the edible plants in our area and also learned how to use them medically.

As time went on I would buy books on the different plants always try to increase my knowledge.

When I went into the army I would always try to learn the different plants in the area and in Germany I learned the flora and fauna that was offered there. In fact when I was in Germany I taught the men under my command how to use the different plants and such if they were put in the position to have to live off the land.

Once I got out of the army I still maintained my interest in learning how to live off the land and also the medicinal uses many plants had.

Fast forward to today and with the outrageous cost of medical treatment, I became our family's first line medical care giver.

I started to expand, learning about all the natural herbs, vitamins and other supplements that are out there.

Nurse Amy of "Doc Bones & Nurse Amy" introduced me to essential oils and I started learning more on how to use them effectively in conjunction with my herbal cures.

Back in 2005 I diagnosed my son's Type 1 Diabetes. Ever article, book and website that I was reading pointed to T1, but did not believe it till I finally told Tracye that we needed to get him to the hospital. From what I could tell he was already in the very dangerous stages of diabetic ketoacidosis.

When we got him to the emergency and I told the nurses what I suspected and congratulated me on making catching it. They said that they see many first time T1 kids already passed out due to DKA.

I want to say that I am not a doctor and I have nothing but the highest respect for doctors and for the things they have to study to stay up to date. I never thought that I had the calling to be a doctor, but I do enjoy the study of folk medicine and the cures and remedies our great grandparents once used. Many of those cures and remedies are making a comeback today.

I think it is very prudent that those of us who are preppers have as much understanding about medicine as we are able. We need to return to having the skills of mending wounds, binding cuts and giving proper first aid.

I think the skill of diagnosing basic illnesses is also something that has been forgotten. It amazes me how many people do not even know the symptoms of a common cold and then rush to the ER thinking they are about to go to their grave.

I have made it a personal responsibility to be the best care giver that I could for the sake of my family.

To this date, whenever we are with our kids and grandkids I am always asked to look at some cut or scratch or help diagnose some belly rumblings, fever or runny nose. In fact my Grandson thinks that if I do not have my flashlight in hand when looking at that splinter, then something must be wrong. No matter what the little prick or scratch, I must look at it with my flashlight so that I can make the proper diagnosis and provide the proper treatment.

Most times it all comes down to a little Neosporin and a band-aid. Sometimes I will use lavender oil or thieves' oil just to help speed the healing. My grandson likes it because it smells good and is "good medicine" not the bad medicine that "tastes yucky".

Today we have Ebola which is trying to break free from the boarders of Africa.

As I sit here writing, I'm hearing a Fox News report about Dr. Kent Brantly, who has just arrived in the US at the university hospital outside of Atlanta.

He is believed to be the first patient with the deadly Ebola virus ever to be treated at a hospital in the United States. He landed at Dobbins Air Reserve Base around 11 a.m. August 2nd, 2014.

The Ebola outbreak that is taking place right now is the largest outbreak in known history.

Past Ebola outbreaks were not as devastating as the current one. I believe that is because this strain of Ebola has mutated in one form or another like many immunosuppressive diseases will over time.

Because our world has gotten smaller due to jet planes flying all over the world, the probability of a virus crossing over into other countries has become much greater.

As with past outbreaks of Ebola, this strain is showing that the virus can live outside the body for up to 10 hours, which increases it's ability to infect people. A victim who is carrying the virus could be walking around in an airport can cough, sneeze, spit, vomit and the virus cells will remain active for up to 10 hours on whatever surface they've landed on.

That is 10 hours that tens if not hundreds of people could come in contact with those virus cells.

Once a person comes into contact with those cells, all they would need to do is touch their mouth, their eye, or scratch an open sore and that person is infected.

The key to living through this is prevention.

Once a family member contracts this horrible disease the outcome is pretty grim. Studies show that there is a 40% chance of survival. 60% of those who contract the disease will die.

If you have not done so, I HIGHLY RECOMMEND that you read my first book, "Survive The Coming Storm – The Value of a Preparedness Lifestyle."

If people are going to truly make it, they will need to self-quarantine and if one does not have enough food, water and other items to ride this storm out, they will have to go out into the public more and more and that is exactly where you do not want to be. To go out into the public means that you will be exposing yourself to Ebola and you will have increased your risk of contracting the disease.

In this book I make MANY recommendations from herbal supplements to OTC medicines. I also make recommendation of getting Hazmat Suits, facemasks, and rubber gloves. At a minimum having a N95 facemask will be a necessity along with bottles of Purell (hand sanitizer) to constantly keep your hands sterile. On top of that all of us will have to break that horrible habit of touching our face, eyes, nose or mouth. Do that during a pandemic and you sign your own death sentence.

If you and your family are not prepared by then, your odds are increased of contracting the deadly Ebola virus. If you are only able to give subpar care to that infected family member, they will probably die and odds are good that others, including you will probably catch the disease.

It is my hope that this book helps you and equips you with information that will help you prepare NOW instead of waiting till the pandemic starts.

You still have time, do what you have to do and even if nothing happens, you have gained valuable supplies that most likely will be needed.

Every 100 years our world suffers a deadly global pandemic. The last killer was the Spanish flu in 1918. In 2018 it will be 100 years from that last deadly pandemic. This makes the "odds" extremely high that a killer pandemic is just around the next corner.

Want to read a real life account?

Read The Hot Zone - http://tinyurl.com/PZ-The-Hot-Zone

Ray Gano
August 5th, 2014

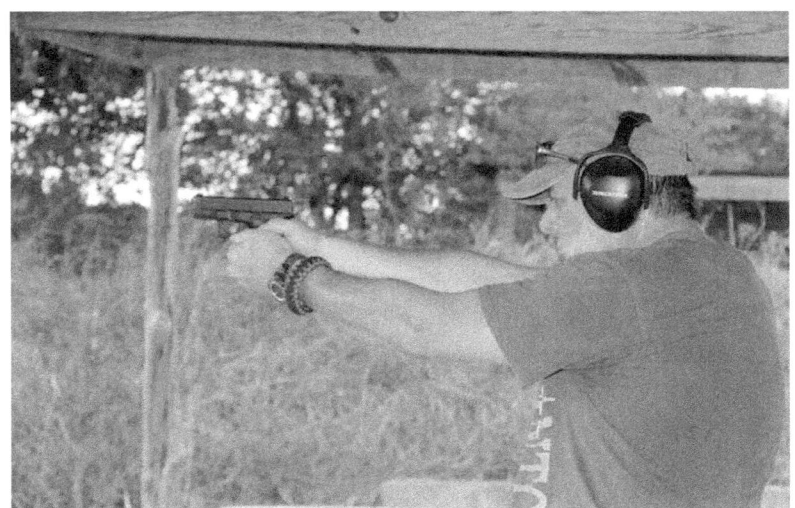
The author shooting his favorite Glock 26

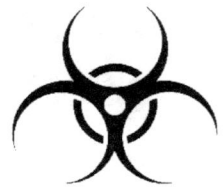

Chapter 1 – Ebola is Here

Matthew 24:7 For nation shall rise against nation, and kingdom against kingdom: and there shall be famines, and pestilences, and earthquakes, in divers places. 8 All these are the beginning of sorrows

The head of the World Health Organization (WHO) Margaret Chan has said "The Ebola outbreak in West Africa is spreading faster than efforts to control it."

She told a summit of regional leaders that failure to contain Ebola could be "catastrophic" in terms of lives lost.

At the time of writing there are over 700 infected people in the North Africa region who have died and more are getting sick daily. Liberia has declared a national state of emergency and countries are locking down their boarders trying to prevent the spread of Ebola to other countries.

Infected Ebola patients are being flown to Atlanta and one has to ask "are health authorities risking a U.S. outbreak?"

CBS News Reported …

> The international Ebola outbreak has caused a wave of alarm among people who are concerned it might spread to their own city or nation. It's a legitimate concern, given that the government of Liberia has already issued a desperate

plea for international help after declaring the pandemic "[beyond] the control of the national government." (1)

I have gotten several emails from people asking if there are any natural cures that can kill Ebola.

At this time there are no proven cures for Ebola, but there are some valuable immune boosting strategies detailed here which can save many lives. Here's what we know so far:

How Ebola spreads

To understand how we need to fight Ebola, we first need to understand how it spreads.

Ebola is a level-4 biohazard virus. It spreads so easily and quickly that even well-trained doctors wearing protective masks and gloves are getting infected from nearby patients. This has been proven by several doctors working in Africa. All of the disease containment protocols were followed and yet, they still got infected.

What the news and popular media is NOT TELLING YOU is that Ebola only needs one single viral organism to enter your body to infect you.

The most common access points for Ebola is through your mouth or eyes.

For example -- A person who rubs their eyes with their finger can instantly become infected with Ebola if a single virus cell was resting on that person's finger.

I was watching FOX News last night and I was absolutely amazed at the incorrect statements they were making about Ebola. One of the main things that are being promoted is that Ebola is not airborne. What the popular media is doing here is splitting hairs.

Ebola can spread through "aerosols," meaning liquid particles suspended in the air. When a person infected with Ebola sneezes, vomits or coughs, they can create Ebola aerosols.

The public health agency of Canada stated the following regarding aerosolized organisms and its association with Ebola…

> "1 - 10 aerosolized organisms are sufficient to cause infection in humans," explains the Public Health Agency of Canada. (2)

This is how Ebola becomes "airborne" even when it is not "traditionally categorized" as an airborne disease.

What are the signs and symptoms of Ebola?

- Fever
- Vomiting
- Diarrhea
- Sore throat
- Joint and muscle aches
- Stomach pain
- Headache
- Measles like rash
- A rash, red eyes, hiccups and Bleeding from body openings may be seen in some patients

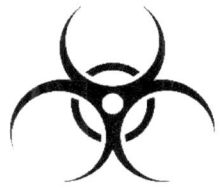

Chapter 2 - Hospitals and a Full Blown Pandemic

Revelation 6:7-8 And when he had opened the fourth seal, I heard the voice of the fourth beast say, Come and see. 8 And I looked, and behold a pale horse: and his name that sat on him was Death, and Hell followed with him. And power was given unto them over the fourth part of the earth, to kill with sword, and with hunger, and with death, and with the beasts of the earth.

As any good doctor will tell you, the majority of today's hospitals is no place for a sick person. That goes double for anyone during a pandemic.

Just take a UV Flashlight into a hospital and you will see blood, urine and other body fluid splatter all over the place.

The idea that hospitals may offer lifesaving solutions during a pandemic where they are able to offer care, heal and rehabilitate, and I hate to say this…is a fairy-tale.

Right now we have two victims who have been flown to Atlanta who will receive top quality care. This will switch from: "Care Giver" mode to: "make the patient comfortable so they can die with as little pain as possible" mode.

I witnessed this personally when there was the H1N1 pandemic in 2009 in New Braunfels Texas.

The same thing happened during the 1918 Spanish flu outbreak.

Today we are a hairs breath away from a pandemic. Be it H1N1 (Spanish Flu), H5N1 (Bird Flu), or the primary topic of this book: Ebola.

Already, major medical associations are backing the idea that home treatment, not hospitalization during a pandemic should be the policy.

The American College of Physicians (ACP), the largest medical-specialty organization and the second-largest physician group in the United States, boasting 119,000 members, released a policy paper entitled... "The Health Care Response to Pandemic Influenza."

You can read it here - http://tinyurl.com/APC-Pandemic-Policy

this short excerpt from their report, backs up what I am saying here...

> *"A pandemic, ACP warns, will place extraordinary and sustained demands on the U.S. health care system. It will require all non-hospital-based health care providers, internists and family practice providers in particular, to be prepared to counsel, diagnose, treat and monitor patients outside of hospital settings in order to decrease the likelihood of surges that would overwhelm hospital capacity."(1)*

As you can see, the proposed plan is very simple, treat the victims as out-patients whenever possible. The responsibility of the infected family member will fall on other family members to provide the needed care and rehabilitation.

This report points out the obvious, that hospitals cannot handle the pandemic load and hospitals WILL COLLAPSE under the onslaught of patients.

This is why I say that hospitals will not be the place to be healed during a pandemic, they will become the place where they are able to control the spread and become the final resting place for anyone being admitted during a pandemic.

Hospital Statistics

When one runs the numbers we can see that there are roughly 900,000 hospital beds in the United States.

At any given time, 95% are already in use.

Here is the kicker, there are only about 105,000 ventilators, and 90% of those are in use. For those of you who do not know, a mechanical ventilator is a machine that makes it easier for patients to breathe until they are able to breathe completely on their own.

Patient suffering from flu or Ebola like symptoms will most likely need a ventilator to help assist in breathing.

> "The US Government estimates that as many as 750,000 people could need a ventilator during a pandemic. Obviously, with only 10,000 or so extra available, 75 people will go without for every person that gets one." (2)

As far as hospital beds are concerned, a moderate pandemic could infect 15 to 30 million Americans at the same time (5% to 10%), and with only 50 thousand extra beds nationwide, the odds of getting into a hospital during a pandemic is almost non-existent.

While some hospitals may try to admit over the maximum number of patients, a breakdown in care will take place, and more and more healthcare providers will in fact contract the disease themselves. Thus needing to be hospitalized, or forced into homecare to be treated by family members also.

Like it or not, the results found in a hospital during a pandemic are not going to be neither very hopeful nor very pretty.

Even in normal times, hospitals are plagued with hospital acquired infections (HAI). During a pandemic this will escalate. Already more than 20,000 Americans die in hospitals from infections which they've contracted at the hospital. This is enough people that the odds are pretty good that you personally know someone, or know some family member or friend of a friend who has contracted a disease or infection while in a hospital.

During a pandemic, those numbers will go through the roof just due to the lack of sanitation procedures to ensure a sterile environment.

Given the staff shortages that will take place, the overcrowding, the growing lack of supplies, AND OH YEA… the lack of ventilators, and the real possibility of contracting a secondary infection in a hospital during a pandemic are very good and very probable.

The standard of care that we are used to in the US would likely vanish overnight. There will be little that a hospital would be able to do for a pandemic patient that couldn't be better done in the home.

Already, FEMA has plans to set up ad-hoc hospitals in high school gymnasiums, community centers, even in some hotels.

But once again, the same problems that hospitals will incur will also take place in those facilities as well, overcrowding, no supplies, lack of sanitation and yes, no ventilators.

These places will become secondary morgues, close behind most hospitals.

This is why I strongly believe that one MUST prepare to treat at home and be able to quarantine one's home so that they can properly care for infected family members.

This is the primary reason I wrote this report / eBook. The time to prepare is before the catastrophic event. If you think that you will be able to get any sort of medical supplies during the onset of a pandemic, let me tell you right here, right now that you are dreaming, and that there will be nothing on the shelves the first moment that FOX News or CNN reports that there are people becoming infected with Ebola, or whatever pandemic disease that might be taking place.

We MUST prepare and we MUST start thinking differently. That is if you and your family are going to make it through this Coming Pandemic Storm.

What you need to do is start getting your home in order. You need to determine what medical supplies you have on hand now and what medical supplies you need to purchase.

PREPAREDNESS TIP – I am not a fan of using Credit Cards. But now is a good time to secure the supplies needed because once a pandemic hits, it will hit like a forest fire being blown by the wind. It will travel and take over in the matter of hours. So, running up your credit card to ensure that you and your family have all the supplies foreseeable that you will need, I believe would be a prudent idea. I would rather worry about paying off a credit card than worry about how many graves I need to dig for family members.

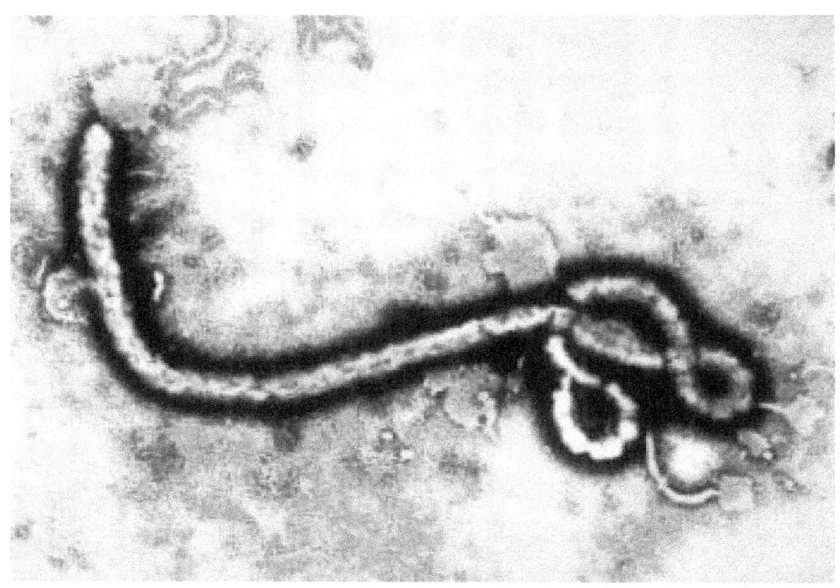

The Ebola Virus

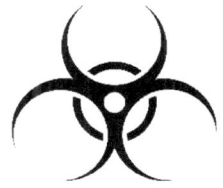

Chapter 3 - Start Thinking Sterile

Exodus 40:31 And Moses and Aaron and his sons washed their hands and their feet thereat:

Sanitizing surfaces is a significant part of any defence against Ebola infections. Studies have proven that that Ebola can be killed with common house hold bleach. It can also be killed using common methyl alcohol – AKA: rubbing alcohol.

Maintaining vigilance is what will set you and your family apart from the common man.

One thing that you can do to start "getting into the sanitary habit" is keeping sanitary wipes with you all the time.

Purell Sanitizing Wipes - http://tinyurl.com/PZ-Sanitizing-Wipes

The sanitizing wipes will help you keep your own hands sterile, but what about surfaces around you? What do you do then? My solution is keeping a small bottle of alcohol spray with you at all times. You can use this to spray door knobs, desk and other flat surfaces that someone may have used, toilet seats, bathroom sink handles, anything that someone else may have touched who may be contaminated with Ebola.

This is why I recommend that you to purchase several refillable bottles so that you can put bleach or ethyl alcohol in them and keep them with you so that you can spray down surfaces or even use them to sanitize your own hands.

Here is a good bottle to purchase -- http://tinyurl.com/PZ-3-5-Refillable-Spray-Bottle

Keeping hand sanitizer all over the home and office where you work is also a very good idea.

Purell Hand Sanitizer with Aloe 8oz - http://tinyurl.com/PZ-Purell-Hand-Sanitizer

You can also purchase Purell hand sanitizer in the large refill bottles. This way you can put it in smaller bottles that you can leave all over the house as well as take with you when you are out and about.

Start Stocking Up on Sanitizing Products

In the past, I've repeatedly recommended stocking up on sanitizing agents as a key preparedness strategy. When "the end of the world as we know it" (TEOTWAWKI) takes place, cleaning supplies will be at a premium. In fact everything will be at a premium. That is why I encourage: buy now.

This is why you need to change the way you think. You need to start looking at things as an investment. The item that you buy today for $3.00 could and most likely will cost $20.00 + when the "poo hits the fan."

Look at things like a stock broker would look at the stock market. The old rule is: "buy low, sell high."

That is what you want to do. By purchasing items now, you are buying at a lower price as compared to the hyper-inflated prices that are inevitable during a pandemic event.

Spray Bottles

One of the best things you can "invest" in is a stock of spray bottles. These are a HUGE help when you are trying to sanitize items and surfaces. Don't buy cheap bottles either; invest in good industrial spray bottles that are made to hold cleaners. You will need these to keep working especially when you need them the most, during a pandemic when you need to sanitize everything and even everyone.

Sprayer Bottles - http://tinyurl.com/PZ-Spray-Bottles

Bleach

One can never have enough bleach. Every home should multiple gallons of bleach on hand. It is inexpensive and easy to store. But one thing that you need to realize is that bottled bleach will lose its effectiveness over time. It is best to use it within one year of purchase to get the "full strength" of the chlorine bleach.

For long term storage, one can buy the chlorine packs that are used to "shock" their pool. Be careful using this though, it is very concentrated and can cause injury.

Pool Shock - http://tinyurl.com/PZ-Pool-Shock

Hydrocide

This is a product that you can pick up at beauty supply / Baber supply shops. It is a germicide that is used to clean scissors, combs, clippers, ect. You can use it on just about any surface. This is where having a good number of spray bottles on hand is a good idea, so that you can have multiple sanitizers that you can use depending on the surface and the situation.

Hydrocide -- http://tinyurl.com/PZ-Hydrocide

Hydrogen Peroxide

This is also a common cleaning / sanitizing agent. It is inexpensive, and you can pick it up cheap at Wal-Mart or any of the other big box stores. Keep multiple bottles on hand. This is also a great item to use for any open cut wounds. It will "fizz" as it reacts to the blood oxidizing and kills germs in the process.

Lugol's Iodine

Iodine is one of the best sanitizers out there. This was once the staple to clean and disinfect medical equipment and many doctor's and dentist offices smelled of it. It's effectiveness on Ebola is not known, but like the other items spoken about; the more of a defence you have, the better. Iodine is also helpful in purifying the blood and is excellent for the thyroid. I use this personally and take about 5-6 drops in a glass of water daily.

Lugol's Iodine - http://tinyurl.com/PZ-Lugols-Iodine

UV Lights In The Home

Using a lot of these cleaners / sanitizers and maintaining a sterile environment in the home is difficult, to almost impossible. One way to battle this is by installing UV lights in portions of the home, like in the Kitchen, possibly the bathroom, and maybe even the laundry room. A UV light helps weaken or even kills most viruses. These areas are where germs and contaminates seem to congregate the most. Having a UV light in each of these areas could help by reducing infection and killing germs.

Sunlight / UV rays kill Ebola. This is probably why you find Ebola more in the tropical / dense population areas, and you don't find it in the desert regions of the world.

If Ebola does make its way to the USA, it would have a higher infectious success rate in places like Florida, Georgia, Louisiana, etc., where the heat and humidity are higher.

UV Light bulb - http://tinyurl.com/PZ-UV-Lightbulb

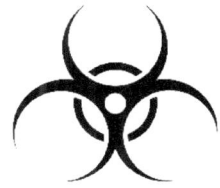

Chapter 4 - Creating a Quarantined Patient Room / Sterile Environment

> Matthew 4:23 And Jesus went about all Galilee, teaching in their synagogues, and preaching the gospel of the kingdom, and healing all manner of sickness and all manner of disease among the people.

This portion of the book is kind of jumping ahead, but this is something that you MUST PLAN FOR. You need to choose a room beforehand so that you know how many supplies you will need, so that you can make this a proper quarantine room.

The first thing you need to determine is: will you be able to create a "clean room" in this bedroom that you will be picking out. The "clean room" is a small space that that you can step in and out of when entering your patient's area. This is usually located at the door which you would normally enter the room from. So this room has to be pretty big and as I have said, the Master Bedroom will be the best room to make into the quarantined patient room.

First thing that you need to do is remove any extra furniture that is NOT necessary. If you have a King / queen bed in this room, exchange it with twin bed or a cot.

You might want to keep a set of drawers in this room so that you can keep all medical supplies, clean rags and towels. Keep anything that you may need to use in there.

A few extra lamps will also be needed as well as tables to store medical supplies on.

I would also recommend some sort of CD player so that the patient can listen to soothing gospel music / audible KJV bible read by Alexander Scorby. The music and scripture will help aid the patient to remain calm and maintain a positive attitude during their battle with the illness.

Creating The "Sterile" Enter / Exit Room

Simply put, you are going to create a small dressing area by taking thick painters plastic that will reach from the ceiling of that room all the way to the floor with a good foot or two of excess that you can then weigh down with sandbags or weights. This will help create a somewhat small, airtight environment where you can enter and exit the patient's room. This room is there so that you can change, decontaminate, and retreat into, if the patient start vomiting or spewing the vomit all over the quarantine room uncontrollably.

Supplies Needed to Create The Clean Room

Clear Thick Painters Plastic (Visqueen) - You can purchase this at home supply stores in rolls. Get multiple rolls so that you have extra on hand. We will need it for walls, floors and you might have to use it for wrapping up a diseased love one. The thicker the plastic is, the better.

Cordless Screw Gun

1.5 – 2 inch long wood screws - approximately 50+ the more the better.

Wooden Yard Sticks / Strips of Wood - approximately 20 + yardsticks. NOTE: if you have a table saw, you can make these by simply cutting down a 2x4 or 2x6. Just cut long strips of the 4 inch / 6 inch side.

Carpenters knife / a very sharp knife to cut the painters plastic.

Sandbags – will hold the excess edges of the plastic down, so that you can create as much of an airtight area as possible.

Common Paper Stapler

Small electric fan

6 Foot ladder

The room needs to have enough space so that you can measure out approximately 4-5 feet square where the door to the room opens. Your quarantine room will need to be rather large in size. In most houses the master bedroom is usually the best because there is usually a bathroom attached. This will enable the patient to use the bathroom without contaminating the rest of the house. The patient may also have to vomit, or have diarrhea. In some cases they may not make it to the bathroom before having to vomit or defecate. This is why you need a large room, so that you can also spread the thick plastic all over to prevent any contaminates from remaining in carpeting or getting on any painted walls. Most master bedrooms will facilitate this.

You are then going to cut sheets of plastic long enough so that you have at least 6 inches of excess that you can roll the plastic onto the wooden yard sticks and then screw these plastic wrapped yard sticks into the ceiling.

You should also have several feet of excess on the floor so that you can use your weights or sandbags to weigh down the plastic. You will want to be careful that your plastic is not too tight. It will eventually rip down from the ceiling if you make it too tight. You want a comfortable amount of excess on the floor so that you can achieve a tight but not too tight plastic sheet wall.

You want to create a large enough area so that you could change into your hazmat suit in this area and still open and close the door to the room. You will want to put a small table and chair there so that you can comfortably change. You need the table to also hold any sort of decontamination supplies you might need when exiting the patient area.

When you have hung all your sheets of plastic, you want to make sure you have a several foot overlap of plastic hanging from ceiling to the floor so that you can create a door. The overlap is to ensure that air from the patient area is not coming in to your "clean room". This is where the small electric fan comes into play. You want the fan to be in your clean area and set on the highest setting that can blow against the overlapped plastic sheet doorway, but not turned up so high that it separates the plastic sheets and exposes you to the air in the patient's room. The forced air is there so that when you enter and exit the patient area, any contaminates will be blown out of the "clean room." That is in best case scenario.

Spread plastic on the walls and on the floor. Wrap 6 inches of plastic around the yardstick and screw them to the tops of the walls allowing the plastic to naturally drape down the wall. If there is a chance of contaminate coming in contact with something that is porous, then put plastic on it. You want to create a room that allows you had to spray it down with bleach or other sanitizer; so it will not soak into the walls or carpet, if necessary. A simple rule of thumb is that if the person is likely to vomit, spit, or defecate on it: cover it.

If you have a King / queen sized bed in the room, pull it out and put in a twin bed or a cot. Place the bed by a window so that sunlight can shine on the patient. The UV rays will help kill the Ebola virus as well as provide light to examine the patient.

Finally, hang plastic around bed in a manner that's still giving you access to the bed. This plastic you are hanging is a "safe wall", so that if you need to, you can run behind it if the patient is about to vomit or defecate. This is a protective barrier like the curtains you see in most hospital rooms. That is why those curtains are there, it isn't to provide privacy to the patient. It is something to duck behind if the patient spews all over the place.

Do NOT enclose the entire bed because you need the patient to have access to clean air.

IF you have forced air / central air / air conditioning you can use that forced air to your advantage. You will need to screen up your windows so that air flow is constantly going out of the window. This will give the patient a fresh supply of clean air and will also push any contaminates out the window. IF you have the means to set up a misting hose outside the window, the mist will then capture any contaminates and cause it to fall to the ground. This helps prevent contaminates from lingering in the air outside the window.

Lastly – remember the UV light bulb, hang it or place it in the ceiling fixture. UV Rays kill the flu and Ebola virus. This is a little extra added insurance that could help prevent others from getting infected as well as the person who is the dedicated care giver.

Added Precaution Regarding the Mattress

If you have plastic mattress covers, put them on the mattress so that the virus does not seep into the mattress itself. You will be forced to discard the mattress if this happens. I would recommend having several of these covers on the bed at the same time so that if the patient vomits or defecates in the bed, you can pull off an outer cover and still have the inner cover protecting the mattress. Have multiple covers on hand so that you do not run out in case there are several accidents of this sort of nature.

You should have a good quarantined patient room ready to occupy, and a "clean room", so that you can enter into the room, change into and out of a hazmat suit, conduct examinations, and the room be reality easy to keep sterile by spraying walls, floors, bathroom areas down with cleanser.

You may want to place a hook or something to hold your hazmat suit in this room. You may also want to keep several bottles of rubbing alcohol in industrial spray bottles and towels so that every time you enter into this room from the patient area, you can spray your liquid resistant hazmat suit down and clean it off from any possible contaminates that might have adhered themselves to the suit while you were in with the patient.

NOW, if you have the money to buy multiple sets of these liquid resistant hazmat suits, then buy as many as you can. You may need them. But try to conserve them as much as possible. This is why I say that you may want to decontaminate the suit with rubbing alcohol before taking it off. The rubbing alcohol kills the Ebola virus and will quickly dry off whereas using a bleach spray may take longer to dry off.

For more information on use of the quarantined patient room, jump to the chapter: "**What Happens If I or Someone Gets Infected?**".

One last thing that you'll want to do is to put some sort of hook lock or means of locking the patient in the quarantine room - but you'll also want to gain access to the room if an emergency arises.

If you have the financial means, it might be wise to purchase a baby video monitor. This will help to reduce repeated exposure to the disease and could help by allowing multiple people to keep an eye on the family member without them actually coming into contact with the patient themselves.

Video Baby Monitor - http://tinyurl.com/PZ-Baby-Video-Monitor

Survival Sick Room with Doc Bone's & Nurse Amy – WATCH NOW >> http://youtu.be/dLmw_nHp63g

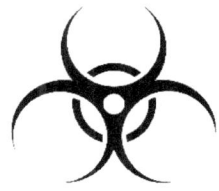

Chapter 5 - My List of Herbal / OTC Supplements That Can Help

> Jeremiah 30:13 There is none to plead thy cause, that thou mayest be bound up: thou hast no healing medicines.

In preparation for a global pandemic, I would stock up on following herbal supplements that have anti-viral properties. There's no proof that these supplements help with the Ebola infections, but because Ebola is an immunosuppressive disease these supplements may help and have had a proven track record having antiviral properties. Ebola is a virus and so it would seem logical of these herbal supplements could help in boosting the immune system and raise one's antibodies.

But the key is to take them at the onset of the disease. The moment that you think that you even MIGHT have come in contact with Ebola, you need to start treating yourself IMMEDIATELY.

These are the very same supplements that I keep on hand all the time.

Sambucol (black elderberry) - http://tinyurl.com/PZ-Sambucol

Colloidal Silver - http://tinyurl.com/PZ-Silver-Sol

Echinacea - http://tinyurl.com/PZ-Echinacea

Propolis - http://tinyurl.com/PZ-Propolis

Ginger Root - http://tinyurl.com/PZ-Ginger-Root

Vitamin C - Rosehips - http://tinyurl.com/PZ-Rosehips

Activated Charcoal - http://tinyurl.com/PZ-Activated-Charcoal

When we lived in Texas, we were in the middle of the H1N1 Swine flu mini pandemic. I got these items as fast as I could and the moment anyone even sniffed, I gave them the following…

- A shot glass of Sambucol (it comes with its own little glass)
- 3-4 sprays of Silver Sol Colloidal silver spray
- 2 caps Echinacea (400 – 500 mg ea)
- 2 caps propolis (1000 mg ea)
- 2 caps ginger root (500 mg ea)
- 2 caps rose hip / vitamin C (500mg ea)
- 1 cap charcoal (280 mg)

This is still the same regiment that I use the moment we feel like some sort of bug is taking hold of our health. To date, we have not contracted any disease or caught the flu when I was proactive with this treatment. This treatment is specifically done to raise one's antibodies and strengthen one's immune system.

Lactic Acid / Naturally Fermented Food's Past Performance of Against The Spanish Flu

Ebola, like the flu, is an immunosuppressive disease. This means that possibly the same treatments and proactive actions one would do to prevent the flu can possibly also be used to prevent the Ebola Virus.

Fermented foods, especially true lactic-acid ferments have been shown to activate the TH-1 immune system and help prevent viral infection.

In societies where lactic acid fermentation is used, studies show that there has been a decrease in the flu associated to these areas.

So, eating and drinking fermented foods regularly may help one prevent illness.

But here is the catch: they have to be homemade. In today's sterile, processed, pasteurized food arena all of the positive probiotics, lactic acid and other health benefits are removed and cooked out.

Some of these lactic acid products that you can make yourself are …

Fermented Milk Products - like yogurt containing lactic-acid bacteria. Studies also show that this may also lower ones risk of allergies.

This is easy to learn to make. If you have an Excalibur dehydrator, you can easily produce your own, cost effectively.

Here is a good video explaining how to do it…

WATCH NOW -- http://youtu.be/EpYwv5E1EXY

Excalibur Dehydrator - http://tinyurl.com/PZ-Excalibur-Dehydrator

Kefir – is similar to a drinking-style yogurt, but it contains beneficial yeast as well as friendly 'probiotic' bacteria found in yogurt. The naturally occurring bacteria and yeast in kefir combine symbiotically to give superior health benefits when consumed regularly. It is loaded with valuable vitamins and minerals and contains easily digestible complete proteins.

Kefir is made from gelatinous white or yellow particles called "grains." This makes kefir unique, because no other milk culture forms grains. These grains contain the bacteria/yeast mixture clumped together with casein (milk proteins) and complex sugars. They look like pieces of coral or small clumps of cauliflower and range from the size of a grain of wheat to that of a hazelnut. Some of the grains have been known to grow in large flat sheets that can be big enough to cover your hand! The grains ferment the milk, incorporating their friendly organisms to create the cultured product. The grains are then removed with a strainer before consumption of the kefir, then added to a new batch of milk. (3)

Homemade Kimchi or Sauerkraut – This is highly beneficial and contains high levels of Lactic Acid. Areas like Eastern Europe, Korea and other areas that eat a lot of fermented cabbage also maintained lower cases of the Spanish Flu.

Making homemade Sauerkraut is very easy and fun to do. In fact here is a video that I produced making my own homemade Sauerkraut using a Harsch Crock Pot. Lactic acid fermentation also produces positive probiotics that help with digestion and promote a healthy digestive track. The juice from this process is also said to help prevent and cure ulcers too

WATCH NOW -- http://youtu.be/ei-mURZpsyl

Harsch Fermination Pot - http://tinyurl.com/PZ-Harsch-10-Liter-Pot

Kombucha Tea - contains probiotic ingredients and has antimicrobial properties. That means it has the power to fight viruses and bacteria. Does that mean kombucha can help the body fight the common cold or flu (influenza) virus? Research and anecdotal evidence suggest that it does, especially when made with green tea.

Kombucha has disease-fighting power

- In *"Kombucha: The Miracle Fungus"*, Harald Tietze states, "Kombucha has the effect of being a natural antibiotic."
- From *Kombucha.org*: "The resulting beverage [kombucha tea] contains dozens of elements, many of which are known to promote healing for a variety of conditions."
- *ChristianMommyBlogger.com* includes green tea kombucha in her "Five Flu-Fighting Foods," due to the catechins in green tea, "more powerful than vitamins C and E..."
- In "Does kombucha provide immunity?" Dr. Arianna Estelle-Symons states: "Green Tea, which has the most readily

available polyphenols has been known for centuries to have some anti-microbial properties. People who drink a lot of Green Tea don't suffer from the 100 or more rhinoviruses as much as people who do not drink Green Tea."

- In 1996 and again 1998, Harmonic Harvest sent out a "Kombucha Questionnaire." Among the health benefits reported by Kombucha drinkers around the world, over 80% reported an increased immunity to colds and flu. (4)

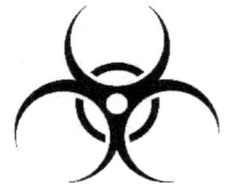

Chapter 6 - Boost Your Immunity – Not Suppress Your Immunity

> Daniel 4:22 it is thou, O king, that art grown and become strong: for thy greatness is grown…

If you have been a reader of mine for some time, you know that I have written about a coming global pandemic for some time now. Like it or not, it is not a matter of "IF", it is a matter of "WHEN"

Historical trends show that a global pandemic takes place approximately every 30 years. A global killer pandemic about every takes place approximately every 100 years. The last global killer was the H1N1 Spanish Flu that killed billions worldwide in the early 1900s. That is about 100 years ago.

With all the poor living choices we have made over the years with chemicals, immune suppressing medications, GMO foods, and the lack of natural vitamins and minerals within our food, one can understand why the odds are very good that we are facing the strong possibility of a killer global pandemic.

With millions upon millions living in high-density metropolis areas and with the growth of air travel over the last 50+ years we can clearly see a "perfect storm" brewing for the spread of infectious disease.

Several years ago there was a very good movie that came out called "Contagion." The plot documents the spread of a virus transmitted through contact, attempts by medical researchers and public health officials to identify and contain the disease, and the loss of social order in a pandemic.

Contagion DVD - http://tinyurl.com/PZ-Contagion-DVD

Depending on the strain, Ebola has a fatality rate of 50 - 90 percent. Studies have shown that 40% of those infected do recover.

Ebola causes severe immunosuppression, and in 60% of the cases it leads to death by internal dehydration by preventing the intestines from absorbing water.

People with suppressed immune systems such as those with AID / HIV, some senior citizens, and some young children seem to be especially vulnerable to Ebola.

This is why a proactive defence strategy is imperative. This is why I support herbal supplements that help increase and support your immune system.

What You Can Do To Stop Suppressing Your Own Immune System

The first line of defence is to help raise your immune system so that your body can fight off any viral attacks that might be presented. But we also need to take steps to stop suppressing our immune system.

How do people suppress their immune systems?

- Lack of sufficient sleep. This is a biggie due to the stressful world with which we live.

- Consumption of processed junk foods and GMOs – Stop eating McDonalds and start cooking healthy locally grown foods. GMOs and junk foods suppress the immune system.

The preservatives in many of these foods are outrageous and are probably the #1 cause of many of the cancers that we have today in our world.

- Stop smoking cigarettes, cigars, marijuana, anything that introduces a foreign substance into the lungs / respiratory system.

- Stop the couch potato lifestyles, get out and exercise.

- Get out in the sun and enjoy nature. UV kills germs, but overdoing it also is harmful. God wants us to live in a balance and not over indulge in anything. Too much of a good thing is harmful.

- Start taking healthy vitamins and minerals.

- Reduce your exposure to pesticides, herbicides, and other harmful chemicals.

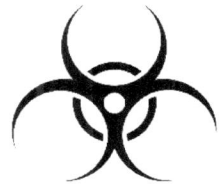

Chapter 7 - What Happens If I or Someone Get Infected?

> Psalms 23:4 Yea, though I walk through the valley of the shadow of death, I will fear no evil: for thou art with me; thy rod and thy staff they comfort me.

With that said; if you believe that you have been infected, one of the first things you need to do is quarantine yourself, so that you'll prevent the possibility of loved ones or others around you from also becoming infected. You do not want to spread the disease.

As I have stated, there is NO KNOW CURE for Ebola. But because it is an immunosuppressive disease, it makes sense to follow many of the same rules you'd follow for other viral infections like the flu, like....

Stay fully hydrated with water and healthy juices. Drink liquids that also help replace electrolytes and other vitamins and minerals that become depleted when one is sick.

Boost your vitamin and supplement intake, give your body the ammunition it needs to help fight this off.

Try to boost your immune system with the supplements mentioned above.

Remain calm and content. A bad attitude helps progress disease; whereas a positive attitude helps the body fight the disease.

Get plenty of rest

Finally... pray and get in God's Word if you are able to still read. If you cannot read I HIGHLY recommend getting CDs / MP3 of Alexander Scorby reading The King James Bible.

Scorby KJV Audio Bible - http://tinyurl.com/PZ-Scorby-Bible-KJV

Hearing God's Word being spoken in the background is helpful no matter what.

As I have said, surviving Ebola is possible. Studies have shown that in some cases and with some strains that a 10%, and up to 50% of people survive Ebola infections.

Studies have NOT shown what these survivors have in common. A positive physiological attitude and belief in God are an advantage. Higher levels of healthy vitamins and minerals may also be a factor. Better, cleaner, peaceful surroundings where a person can properly rehabilitate might have something to do with it. No matter what it is, to date, studies have not been able to identify the common factor.

With all of our medical knowledge, technology, know-how and skill, we still do not have a cure for the Ebola Virus. Pretty much the only treatment is the use of anti-viral drugs at the early onset of the disease. The rest of the approach is a "wait and see" Either the person recovers or they do not.

All we can do is take action in prevention and by being proactive with our health.

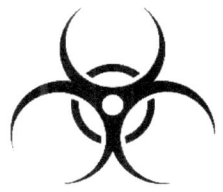

Chapter 8 - After The Infection – Things Will Be Hard To Find

> 2 Kings 6:25 And there was a great famine in Samaria: and, behold, they besieged it, until an ass's head was sold for fourscore pieces of silver, and the fourth part of a cab of dove's dung for five pieces of silver.

IF Ebola does strike all the items I have mentioned will fly off the shelves within hours. We will see social unrest and quite possibly riots.

Other things that you can add that will be VERY HARD TO FIND if there is a pandemic, are the following...

N95 masks - that filter out all bacteria and viruses. Supplies of N95 masks will become depleted during an influenza, pandemic or wide-spread outbreaks of other infectious respiratory illnesses. Have these on hand so that IF someone in your family becomes ill with Ebola, you will be able to treat them without inhaling the virus.

N95 masks - http://tinyurl.com/PZ-N95-Masks

Non-latex disposable gloves – Like the masks, these too will be far and few in between. Putting a protective barrier between you, another possibly contaminated object and possibly infected individuals will become critical. Disposable Nitril Gloves will become a mainstay.

Non-latex disposable gloves - http://tinyurl.com/PZ-disposable-gloves

Liquid Repellent Suits – AKA: Hazmat suits, may be needed, and will in fact be needed if you need to treat a family member in the home. These suits provide that extra protective barrier that you will need if have to come in contact with an ill family member or even have to go into "hot zones"

Liquid Repellent Suits - http://tinyurl.com/PZ-Liquid-Repellent-Suits

Paper Gowns - are also something that should be stocked up on. They can be quickly changed and are quickly disposable. They are NOT a long term wearing solution, but a good solution when one needs to come in contact with an infected family member so that they can check in on the patient, check symptoms, help with food or drink, (something quick like this).

Paper Gowns - http://tinyurl.com/PZ-Paper-Gowns

Medical Treatment Tools

Electronic Ear Thermometer – NO ORAL - http://tinyurl.com/PZ-Electronic-Ear-Thermometer

Automatic Blood Pressure Monitor - http://tinyurl.com/PZ-Blood-Pressure-Monitor

Stethoscope - http://tinyurl.com/PZ-Stethoscope

Tongue Depressors - http://tinyurl.com/PZ-Tongue-Depressors

Medical Eye Goggles - http://tinyurl.com/PZ-Medical-Eye-Goggles

Fenix Flashlight – five brightness levels - http://tinyurl.com/PZ-Fenix-PD35-Flashlight

Purell Hand Sanitizer with Aloe 8oz - http://tinyurl.com/PZ-Purell-Hand-Sanitizer

Notebook for recording vital signs & keeping patient notes

Over The Counter Medicines You Need To Keep On Hand

Any medicines that fight the flu will also become harder and harder to find as well as any supplies associated to the Flu.

Because the Flu is an immunosuppressive disease like Ebola, the following OCT medicines will also become harder and harder to find.

Medicines like …

Bayer Aspirin – http://tinyurl.com/PZ-Bayer-Aspirin

Extra Strength Tylenol - http://tinyurl.com/PZ-Extra-Strength-Tylenol

Children's Tylenol - http://tinyurl.com/PZ-Childrens-Tylenol

Boiron Oscillococcinum – http://tinyurl.com/PZ-Oscillococcinum

Cold-Eeze Immune Support - http://tinyurl.com/PZ-Cold-Eze

Thieves Oil - http://tinyurl.com/PZ-Thieves-Oil

Vicks Nyquil Cold & Flu Daytime & Nighttime – http://tinyurl.com/PZ-Vicks-Nyquil

Quantum Health Thera Zinc Spray - http://tinyurl.com/PZ-Zinc-Spray

Benadryl 25mg capsules - 1 tablet every 4 hours as needed for nasal congestion, allergy, or itching if applicable - http://preview.tinyurl.com/PZ-Benadryl

Tums Ex - http://tinyurl.com/PZ-Tums-Ex\

Caffeinated Tea – Helps relieve headache - http://tinyurl.com/PZ-Caffeinated-Tea

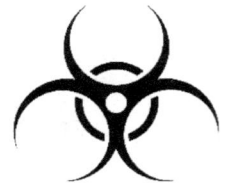

Chapter 9 - Preventing and Identifying Dehydration – The #1 Killer

Psalm 63:1 O God, thou art my God; early will I seek thee: my soul thirsteth for thee, my flesh longeth for thee in a dry and thirsty land, where no water is;

This book has been a major contributor in our family's pandemic preparations. I HIGHLY recommend you get this, print it out and keep it in a binder.

You can download this incredible book at: http://prophezine.com/media/com_acymailing/upload/the_coming_flu_pandemic.pdf

The primary way that Ebola kills is that it dehydrates the victim. This is why preventing dehydration in your loved one will be more effective than all of the other treatments combined.

When people suffer from a fever or have diarrhea, they lose mass amounts of water. This is why knowing and treating for dehydration is very important.

Symptoms of Dehydration

Mild to moderate dehydration is likely to cause:

- Dry, sticky mouth

- Sleepiness or tiredness — children are likely to be less active than usual
- Thirst
- Decreased urine output
- No wet diapers for three hours for infants
- Few or no tears when crying
- Dry skin
- Headache
- Constipation
- Dizziness or light-headedness

Severe dehydration, a medical emergency, can cause:

- Extreme thirst
- Extreme fussiness or sleepiness in infants and children; irritability and confusion in adults
- Very dry mouth, skin and mucous membranes
- Little or no urination — any urine that is produced will be darker than normal
- Sunken eyes
- Shrivelled and dry skin that lacks elasticity and doesn't "bounce back" when pinched into a fold
- In infants, sunken fontanels — the soft spots on the top of a baby's head
- Low blood pressure
- Rapid heartbeat
- Rapid breathing
- No tears when crying
- Fever
- In the most serious cases, delirium or unconsciousness

Unfortunately, thirst isn't always a reliable gauge of the body's need for water, especially in children and older adults. A better indicator is the color of your urine: Clear or light-colored urine means you're well hydrated, whereas a dark yellow or amber color usually signals dehydration. (5)

A very quick test to see of dehydration is present is to pinch the skin on the back of the patients hand and pull it upwards being careful not to cause pain.

Release the skin and if the "bump" from the pinch remains, the person is severely dehydrated and needs to get fluids in them right away.

If you believe that dehydration is present you need to start giving the person fluids by mouth.

By this point I am assuming that your family member is in the home and you need to take care of them. So you will not have access to modern medical supplies and unless you are doctor, nurse or EMT, you will not have the experience to put in an Intravenous drip line.

.If the patient is too ill to drink, someone will have to sit with the patient giving him or her fluids drop by drop if needed. Using a turkey baster is a good solution.

Easy Reach Baster - http://preview.tinyurl.com/PZ-Easy-Reach-Baster

You'll want to continue giving the loved one liquid, drop by drop 'till maybe they can then take a teaspoon of liquids.

It is critical that you don't stop until the patient has been able to keep down at least quart of fluids. This will probably take several hours, so be patient. This is also why you will need to have the liquid repellent hazmat suit so that you can spend hours with the patient if need be.

Keeping the person hydrated will have a dramatic effect on their wellbeing. Believe it or not, this very simple and time consuming thing quiet possibly will save that loved one's life.

If the patient is able to urinate, this is a good prognostic sign and when this happens you can assume you have restored their hydration back to a safer level.

Please understand that "Safer" should not be confused with safe.

The person can quickly become dehydrated again just by sweating from the fever, diarrhea, or vomiting.

You need to continue "pushing the fluids," so don't let your guard down.

IF the family member has a high fever they should probably not be given hot fluids because it will raise the temperature further.

Simple common sense should tell you that if the loved one is hot with fever they will probably prefer cool or even a cold beverage. If it is cold outside especially if the patient is cold, the person could probably use hot fluids. Situation will dictate with this. The better you know the person you are caring for, the better care you can give.

Keeping the person you are caring for hydrated will be one of the main activities day in and day out, until the crisis passes.

Try and get a minimum of 2 to 3 quarts of fluids down the patient every day.

Don't give up or slack off.

Make this your most important task.

NOTE – I wanted to endorse the book "Preparing for the Coming Flu Pandemic" by Grattan Woodson MD, FACP. His information helped immensely with this past chapter. I will provide a link to the PDF book in the LINKS portion at the end.

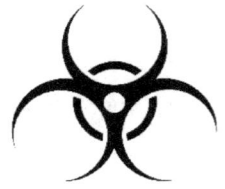

Chapter 10 - Preventing The Virus From Spreading Within The Household

It is unlikely that we will be able to limit exposure to the virus if there are a lot of sick people around us or in the home where we are treating people.

What we must do as the caregiver is **be ever vigilant and make staying decontaminated the utmost priority**.

If we as the caregiver fall to this disease, who will care for us?

So it is imperative that we operate in as much of a sterile environment as we are able to maintain.

Ebola is HIGHLY contagious and is easily passed from one person to the next. This, in and of itself, is difficult to control even in the hospital setting. Doing this in a home setting makes things even more difficult, BUT IT IS NOT IMPOSSIBLE.

We can be good caregivers if we **stay alert and maintain proper quarantine procedures**.

Keep a Record on Every Patient

It will be very useful for you to write down certain information about the patient, or patients you are taking care of at home. Devote a section of the notebook to each patient you are taking care of. Keep the record in chronological order day by day. Keep as accurate and careful records as you can. Don't worry about keeping a perfect record; just keep one that is good enough.

Each day start with the patient's vital signs. Include their temperature, pulse rate, breathing rate, and blood pressure. Repeat the vital signs routinely 4 times daily (for instance at 0800, 1200, 1600, and 2000). These vital signs should be measured more often in very sick patients. You can get a really clear picture of how the patient is doing using these simple measurements.

It is very important to keep up with the patient's fluid intake and their output so record the fluid they are taking in and passing out in a notebook. Intake is pretty easy since you are giving them the fluids but output can be difficult to accurately record. Have the patients to save all their urine by urinating in a bucket, pot, or basin instead of the toilet. Measure the urine output using the kitchen-measuring cup. The amount taken in is always more than the amount passed out because of the insensible losses described above (loss through the skin and in the breath). If the patient is incontinent of urine, just indicate in the record that the patient was incontinent of a small, medium or large amount of urine. For our purposes, large is good, small is bad.

HOME PATIENT RECORD

Name of
patient_____

_____

Name of healthcare
provider_____

_____

Date	Time	Observations*	Temperature	Medication

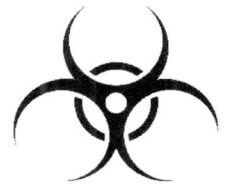

Chapter 11 - Dealing With The Sanitation Issues of Your Quarantined Patient Room

Cleaning and disinfecting are your main weapons when it comes to preventing infectious diseases like Ebola from spreading.

1. Know the difference between cleaning, disinfecting, and sanitizing

Cleaning

Cleaning removes the germs, dirt, and other undesired substances from surfaces and or objects.

Simply put. Cleaning works by using soap (or detergent) and water to physically remove germs, debris, dirt from the surfaces.

NOTE - This process does not necessarily kill germs, but by removing them, it lowers their numbers and possibly lowers the risk of spreading the virus/infection.

Disinfecting

Disinfecting kills germs on surfaces or objects by using chemicals to kill the germs on them. A good example of a simple disinfectant is Lysol Spray. Lysol has an "anti-flu – anti-bacterial" formula in different scents that not only make the room smell good but will also disinfect the area.

Lysol Spray – http://tinyurl.com/PZ-Lysol-Spray

NOTE - This process does not necessarily clean dirty surfaces or remove germs, but it kills the remaining germs that might be left over after cleaning.

This is why it is important to **clean**, and **then disinfect**. This will help to kill any leftover germs that might be lingering **after the cleaning process**. Doing **both** of these will lower the risk of possibly spreading the Ebola virus.

Sanitizing

The process of doing both **cleaning** and **disinfecting combined** is also known as: "**Sanitizing**."

2. Clean and disinfect surfaces and objects that are touched often

When handling patients, there are areas and items that are frequently touched. These are the areas you want to focus on when you are sanitizing the room. Objects and areas touched often are…

- ALL flat surfaces
- Desks & Tabletops
- Countertops
- Nightstands
- Doorknobs,
- Sinks and Faucet Handles
- Toilets, and Toilet handles
- Showers & Bathtubs and their faucet handles
- All wall mounted light switch and plates
- Phones if they are present in the room.
- Radio and TV remotes

- Finally - Immediately clean ANY surfaces and objects that are visibly soiled with any sort of body fluids.

3. Create a routine / cleaning list

It is Important maintain a routine / cleaning list. You may forget to clean and disinfect an area on one day, and then the other days remember to clean and disinfect those areas.

You must maintain consistency so that virus germs do not linger. The Ebola virus is known to continue to be infectious for up to 10 hours on its own outside the body.

Most studies have shown that the flu virus can also live and potentially infect a person for only 2 to 8 hours outside the body.

Ebola and Flu viruses are relatively fragile, so standard cleaning and disinfecting practices are sufficient to remove or kill them.

4. Clean and disinfect correctly

First and foremost, if you are using any sort of commercial cleaner; follow the label's directions as they apply to that particular cleaning and disinfecting product. Wash surfaces with a general household cleaner to remove germs. Rinse with water, and **then follow up with your disinfectant** to kill germs.

IF you do not have any commercial pre-mixed disinfectant then the best option is using FRESH chlorine bleach solution. You will want to use FRESH because bleach will lose its chemical properties over time. A good rule of thumb is to not use bleach that is over a year old. Most bleach purchased at the store will have an expiration date, or a date when it was manufactured.

How to make a bleach disinfectant solution:

Add 1 tablespoon of bleach to 1 quart (4 cups) of water. For a larger supply of disinfectant, add ¼ cup of bleach to 1 gallon (16 cups) of water.

Apply the solution to the surface with a cloth or with a spray bottle.

Let it stand for 3 to 5 minutes.

Wipe the surface down and then rinse with clean water.

NOTE – To properly disinfect, it usually requires the bleach solution to remain on the surface for a certain period of time (3 to 5 minutes).

NOTE – Use disinfecting wipes on electronic items that are touched often, such as phones and computers.

Lysol Wipes - http://tinyurl.com/PZ-Lysol-Wipes

Pay close attention to the directions for using disinfecting wipes. You may need to use more than one wipe to keep the surface wet for the stated length of contact time. Make sure that the electronics can withstand the use of liquids for cleaning and disinfecting.

Wash and dry bed sheets, towels, and other linens as you normally do with household laundry soap. Adding some bleach to the load will also help disinfect. HANG/CLOTHSLINE DRY the linens, the UV light from the sun will also kill the Ebola virus.

ALL eating utensils and dishes that the patient has used need to also be properly cleaned and disinfected. Run a sink of hot water and add some bleach to the water. Let these items soak for a while to ensure that all germs and virus are killed.

Linens used by patient should be cleaned separately, and they should NOT be shared unless they've been washed thoroughly and disinfected.

Finally, wash your hands with soap and water and then use Purell/Hand Sanitizer for extra insurance after handling soiled dishes, clothes, or laundry items that were used by the patient.

Purell Hand Sanitizer with Aloe 8oz - http://tinyurl.com/PZ-Purell-Hand-Sanitizer

5. Use products safely

One thing that you need to do is pay close attention to the warning labels and directions when using the product.

DO NOT MIX CLEANING PRODUCTS – ESPECIALLY BLEACH AND AMONIA.

These items when mixed create a **deadly gas** that **can kill if inhaled**.

It is good procedure when cleaning any items used by the patient; you should be using your mask, goggles and heavy duty gloves. If you use bleach over a span of time, it will cause sores on the hands (if gloves are not worn). So, make sure that you always use gloves to protect your hands when working with any bleach solutions.

6. Handle Waste Properly

Follow procedure when handling waste. If In doubt, bag infected items that are to be disposed of in multiple plastic bags. You should be wearing full protective clothing when coming in direct contact with any infected waste.

Have "no-touch" waste bins / trash cans in the area where the patient is located. Use this "no-touch" garbage can just for the disposal of contaminated items: disposable cleaning items used to clean surfaces, used rags, paper gowns should be placed in the "no-touch" bin/ trash can immediately after you use them. When you are emptying these "no-touch" bins and trashcans, avoid touching anything inside of the bins/trashcans. If there is anything you are using to clean with and it is disposable; then dispose of it.

Again, wash your hands with soap and water after emptying waste baskets, or anything that may have come in contact with contaminated items.

Cleaning Items You May Need For Your Quarantined Patient Room

Cloth Towels - http://tinyurl.com/PZ-Cotton-Towels

Paper Towels - http://tinyurl.com/PZ-Paper-Hand-Towels

Spray bottles of cleaning solution / disinfectant

Mops, buckets and pre-made cleaning / disinfectant solution just in case you need to take care of a quick clean up.

Commercial 50-Gallon Recycling Rollout Trash Can W/ Lid - http://tinyurl.com/PZ-50gal-Trashcan-with-lid

13 Gallon "Blackout" Garbage Bags - http://tinyurl.com/PZ-Blackout-Bags-13gal

30 Gallon Hefty "rip resistant" / Stretch Garbage bags - http://tinyurl.com/PZ-Rip-Resistant-30gal-Bags

55 Gal Trash Bags - http://tinyurl.com/PZ-55-Gal-Trash-Bags

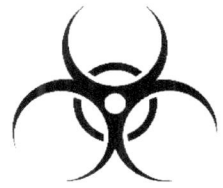

Chapter 12 - Dealing with Death, and Proper Disposal of the Loved One's Body

> John 11:14 Then said Jesus unto them plainly, Lazarus is dead.

As disturbing as this is, it is a topic that I have to cover. It is: dealing with the dead. It is going to be one of **the most difficult things to deal with** if we are hit with a pandemic. Already we are seeing in North Africa how the large numbers of deaths are affecting the populace.

Worse than that, because the bodies are not being disposed of properly, family members are "washing" and coming into contact with contaminates. This is causing the disease to affect more and more people.

Just in the few days spent writing this book, the death toll has risen from 700, to over 875 people dead due to this Ebola outbreak taking place in North Africa.

History proves that a pandemic, natural disaster or terrorist event will in fact overwhelm the local response systems in place which normally care for the deceased. What happens is that the responsibility falls on the local community.

Odds are that if you are reading this you probably do not have experience in dealing with mass fatalities, planning and disposal of the dead. Because **most of us do not have that experience** this amplifies the problems, like we are seeing first-hand in North Africa.

All of this results in the mismanagement of human remains.

Dealing with the dead is critical, just in the fact, how they are treated will have long lasting effect on the surviving family members.

Correct ID needs to be taken into account, so that legal issues of inheritance, insurance, probate, etc, can be also taken care of properly.

Risk to The Body Handlers

Like those who will be care givers, those in charge of handling the human remains have a high risk of coming into contact with body fluids, feces and natural leakage that takes place as a body starts to decompose.

On top of dealing with the Ebola virus these individuals may have to also be concerned with…

- Hepatitis B and C
- HIV
- Tuberculosis
- Diarrheal disease

All of these diseases live upon and within the blood, which is often mixed with the other body fluids upon death.

Safety Precautions For The Body Handlers

In most cases of natural disaster and terrorist events, basic hygiene will protect the workers from exposure to diseases spread by blood and certain body fluids. But we are not talking about these sorts of events. People will be tasked in dealing with people who died from Ebola. Ebola can still be spread even when the person is dead. So, the precautions that are taken to keep the care giver safe are the very same precautions that those tasked with disposing of the body will have to take.

Like those who are care givers the body handlers will need to use the same protective coverings while coming in contact with the infected dead.

- Liquid resistant Hazmat suits.
- Use rubber gloves and boots
- N95 face masks & proper goggles to protect the eyes

Note on wearing gloves: Get into the habit of wearing two sets of gloves, the inner set AND the outer set.

This way, when you take off your hazmat suit, boots and first set of gloves you still have gloves on to protect you from your mask and goggles which might be infected. Once you have taken off the mask and goggles, you can then, pull the gloves off, and as you are pulling them off, allow them to be turned inside out. This way, when you handle the glove, you are handling the part that was next to your skin and not what was exposed to the mask and goggles.

When donning your hazmat suit, duct tape around boots and gloves so that the virus cannot gain access though one of these openings. Yes it is true, **the world is held together with duct tape.**

It would be highly advisable: if someone has **any sort of open sore or wound**, they should be allowed to heal up before dealing with the dead. Open sores or wounds are a means for the virus to enter the body. Because the person will be busy working and thinking about the "normal" means for the virus to enter (i.e. mouth, nose, eyes), they may not be thinking about an open sore or wound. So, risk of infection for people with open wounds and sores needs to be taken into consideration and they may possibly need to be re-tasked with other chores that do not allow them to come into contact with the infected victims or the infected dead.

When finished with the job of disposing of the infected dead, decontamination procedures need to be strictly adhered to.

Before entering a clean area one needs to be sprayed down with bleach solution or alcohol solution. Using a common garden sprayer filled with the proper decon solution is a good idea.

Garden Sprayer - http://tinyurl.com/PZ-Garden-Sprayer

Once the person is completely sprayed down, they can then enter a first stage "clean area" where they can then disrobe from their outer hazmat suit, gloves, and boots.

DO NOT TAKE OFF YOUR MASK OR GOGGLES FIRST!!!

This seems to be the natural thing for most people to do. But it is just good practice to not take off the mask and goggles until one's entire suit, boots and first layer of gloves are taken off.

Once all of these items are properly taken off and put in a hazmat container; **then** one can take off the mask and gloves and proceed to further decontamination.

At this point make sure the worker washes their hands with soap and water. It is good practise to also use Purell after that initial washing.

Still avoid wiping face or mouth with hands. Use only clean sterile towels to take care of this.

Equipment & Vehicle Decontamination & Personnel

Infection may also spread through contact with the dirty clothing or bed linens from a patient with Ebola. Disinfection is therefore required, before handling these items.

Wash and disinfect all equipment, clothes, and vehicles used for transporting the bodies by using boiling water and bleach solution for small items, clothes, tools and anything that can be hand-washed.

Use the garden sprayer with a bleach solution and spray all of the equipment down thoroughly. Do not miss any spots that are too large to wash in boiling water and bleach solution.

People in charge of cleaning up equipment should have more industrial grade protection. For example: heavy duty rubber gloves will help protect from the scalding water and over exposure to the bleach solution. Having an N95 painters mask is also a good idea, since they will be doing more vigorous work cleaning up equipment. It is also wise to put these workers in heavy duty rain suits that will stand up to the water, bleach and the other cleaning solutions being used.

Heavy Duty Rain Suit - http://tinyurl.com/PZ-Heavy-Duty-Rain-Suit

Heavy Duty Rubber Gloves - http://tinyurl.com/PZ-Heavy-Duty-Rubber-Gloves

N95 Painters Mask - http://tinyurl.com/PZ-Painter-N95-Mask

Heavy Duty Work Boots - http://tinyurl.com/PZ-Heavy-Duty-Work-Boots

Wrap duct tape around the openings were gloves and suit, and boot and suit come in contact to prevent liquids from entering under the suit. Running a few strips of duct tape down the front where the jacket and pants open and close is also a good procedure.

Actual Body Recovery

Body recovery is the first step in managing infected dead. This could be as "easy" as getting a deceased family member out from a room where they've died, or having to recover bodies from pastures, allies, vacant lots, inside of vehicles, just about anywhere someone could die.

The more we have planned for this event, the less chaotic and disorganized it will be.

You see, the recovery is critical. The body is still infected and **can still spread infection**. The moment the person dies body fluids start to pool and gravity takes effect. Within minutes to hours after death the deceased body will release urine and feces. Just like when the person was alive, these fluids are just as infectious. So the faster the dead body can be dealt with, the faster body fluids are stopped from passing on the Ebola virus.

Within hours to days, the body will start to seriously decompose. If temperatures are high, this process will be faster. So it is imperative to act quickly. It is during this time frame that methane gasses will start to grow causing the body to bloat and expand. In some cases if the gasses are not allowed to exit, the dead body will literally explode. This will cause infectious body fluids and the virus to be spread all over the area where the dead body was located.

To get an idea of what this could be like, here is a video of a dead whale exploding...

Exploding sperm whale carcass caught on camera in the Faroe Islands - http://youtu.be/7X0hq0ug9q4

So, one can see that it only takes a matter of days and heat for a dead body to quickly decompose. Time is critical before a situation gets worse and causes the risk factor for the Ebola virus to be a lot higher.

Burial & Cremation – Per: The World Health Organization Website

Burial

Burial is the preferred method of body disposal in emergency situations, unless there are cultural and religious observances which prohibit it.

The location of graveyards should be agreed upon with the community, and attention should be given to ground conditions, proximity to groundwater drinking sources (which should be a least 50m) and to the nearest habitat (500m). An area of at least 1500m2 per 10,000 (population) is required. The burial site can be divided to accommodate different religious groups if necessary.

Burial depth should be at least 1.5m above the groundwater table, with at least a 1m covering of soil.

Burial in individual graves is preferred and can be dug manually.

If coffins are not available, corpses should be wrapped in plastic sheeting to keep the remains separate from the soil. Burial procedures should be consistent with the usual practices of the community concerned.

Cremation

There are no health advantages of cremation over burial but some communities may prefer it for religious or cultural reasons.

Factors against it are the amount of fuel required by a single cremation (approx 300kg. wood) and the smoke pollution caused.

For this reason, cremation sites should be located at least 500m downwind of dwellings.

The resultant ashes should be disposed of according to the cultural and religious practice of the community. (6)

If an Ebola pandemic is taking place. The odds are good that local communities will have some area dedicated to the disposal of dead bodies.

If you live in the country and community burial sites are not accessible, then you are going to have to find a proper place to dispose of the body. As mentioned above you need to take into consideration ground water, areas where livestock may congregate as well as dealing with coyotes, dogs, wolves or other animals that may dig up the body.

NOTE - If this happens, Ebola is contagious to dogs and other animals in the canine family, and this can turn into another source of transmitting the disease.

If you have to bury a body, ensure that you place rocks and other heavy items over the grave site so that these animals will not be able to dig them up.

Keeping Records During The Body Collection Process

With the legal world we live in, it is important that we keep records of the person who dies.

It is a good idea to take several pictures of the deceased so that proper ID can be made. All medical records that were being kept should also be included in the death records.

Time of death and witnesses should also be recorded. Anything that will help the family prove death, and help in any legal, insurance or inheritance issues, should be included.

If the person provided a last will and testament on their deathbed: An audio tape or video tape of the person's wishes could also help the family in dealing with these legal issues.

It is safe to say that the more records you are able to create and keep while giving care and at the time of death, the more it will help the family, in the long run.

Dead Body Identification Form

Body/Body Part (B/BP) Code:

(Use unique numbering and include on associated files, photographs or stored objects.)

Possible identity of
body:_____

Person Reporting
Name:_____

Official Status: Place &
Date:_____

Signature:_____

_____

Recovery Details (Include place, date, time, by whom, and circumstances, including name and possible relationship)

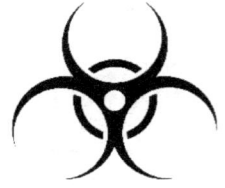

Chapter 13 - Conclusion

It is my hope and desire that the events in the book do not come to fruition; I pray that this Ebola outbreak will just "fizzle out" and that the world will be safe from this killer virus.

But, as I have said, historically speaking the world is due its 100 year pandemic. 1918 was the last one that took place.

History is not linear, history is cyclical. I say that because King Solomon stated something very wise and profound.

> Ecclesiastes 1:9-11
>
> 9 The thing that hath been, it is that which shall be; and that which is done is that which shall be done: and there is no new thing under the sun.
>
> 10 Is there any thing whereof it may be said, See, this is new? it hath been already of old time, which was before us.
>
> 11 There is no remembrance of former things; neither shall there be any remembrance of things that are to come with those that shall come after.

In other words we forget our history and the events of our past. Many choose to not learn from our history and because of that, make the same mistakes those before us made as well.

No matter what, some sort of pandemic **is coming**. We have a chance to get ready. Just look at Noah, the original "dooms-day prepper." Do you think being on that ark for 320 days was like being on Carnival Cruise Line ship? No, it stank, everyone was probably getting sea sick, and cleaning up all those messes and the list goes on. What we learn is that Noah made it through the storm with himself and his family alive and in good health. We can do that same thing; we just have to prepare our own arks.

At a minimum we need to have at a bare bones minimum is 90 days of food, water and any other critical items that you or your family use on a regular basis.

Why 90 days?

Because it takes man at least 90 day to get used to his new normal and start adapting. If you are able to ride out this period when it is the most unstable, you will do well.

But to do that, you have to prepare.

You still have time; start building your ark now.

You will be glad about heeding my call to prepare, and your family will be glad as well.

Finally, here is what scripture says...

> 1 Timothy 5:8 But if any provide not for his own, and specially for those of his own house, he hath denied the faith, and is worse than an infidel.

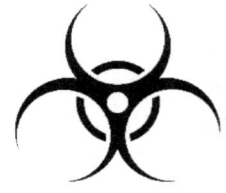

Chapter 14 – Recommended Websites

WHO Ebola Fact Sheet -
http://www.who.int/mediacentre/factsheets/fs103/en/

CDC Ebola Fact Sheet - http://www.cdc.gov/vhf/ebola/

Prophezine – http://www.prophezine.com

Economic Collapse - http://theeconomiccollapseblog.com

The Servant Warrior - www.theservantwarrior.com

Survival 4 Christians - http://survival4christians.blogspot.com

Doom & Bloom – Doc Bones – Nurse Amy -
http://www.doomandbloom.net

The Survival Mom - http://thesurvivalmom.com

Ray Gano's Facebook - https://www.facebook.com/RayGano

Prophezine's Facebook -
https://www.facebook.com/groups/prophezine/

The Servant- Warrior Facebook -
https://www.facebook.com/groups/theservantwarrior/

E-sword – GREAT Free Bible Program - http://www.e-sword.net

Here are 11 ebooks that will be helpful in an Ebola / Flu Pandemic situation, including – "Where There Is No Doctor" and the ebook "Preparing for the Coming Flu Pandemic"

Click on the following URL

http://www.prophezine.com/images/stories/TEOTWAWKI/EBOLA.zip

Appendix A

25 Critical Facts About This Ebola Outbreak That Every American Needs To Know

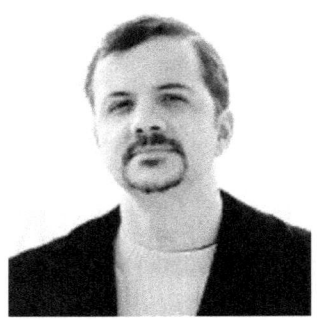

By Michael Snyder

What would a global pandemic look like for a disease that has no cure and that kills more than half of the people that it infects? Let's hope that we don't get to find out, but what we do know is that more than 100 health workers that were on the front lines of fighting this disease have ended up getting it themselves. The top health officials in the entire world are sounding the alarm and the phrase "out of control" is constantly being thrown around by professionals with decades of experience. So should average Americans be concerned about Ebola? If so, how bad could an Ebola outbreak in the U.S. potentially become? The following are 25 critical facts about this Ebola outbreak that every American needs to know...

#1 As the chart below demonstrates, the spread of Ebola is starting to become exponential...

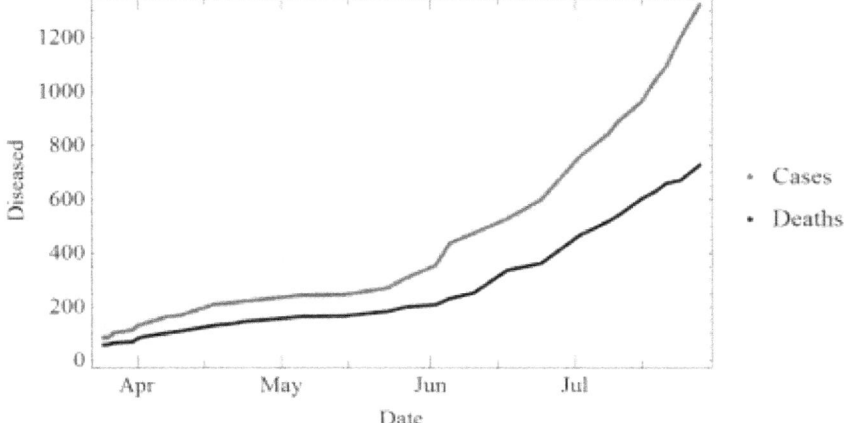

#2 This is already the worst Ebola outbreak in recorded history by far.

#3 The head of the World Health Organization says that this outbreak "is moving faster than our efforts to control it".

#4 The head of Doctors Without Borders says that this outbreak is "out of control".

#5 So far, more than 100 health workers that were on the front lines fighting the virus have ended up contracting Ebola themselves. This is happening despite the fact that they go to extraordinary lengths to keep from getting the disease.

#6 There is no cure for Ebola.

#7 The death rate for this current Ebola outbreak is over 50 percent, and experts say that it can kill "up to 90% of those infected".

#8 The incubation rate for Ebola ranges from two days to 21 days. Therefore, someone can be carrying it around for up to three weeks without even knowing it.

#9 For the first time ever, human Ebola patients are being brought to the United States. And as Paul Craig Roberts so aptly put it the other day, all it would take is "one cough, one sneeze, one drop of saliva, and the virus is loose".

#10 This has already potentially happened in the United Kingdom. A woman reportedly collapsed and later died on Saturday after she got off of a flight from Sierra Leone at Gatwick Airport.

#11 A study conducted in 2012 proved that Ebola could be transmitted between pigs and monkeys that were in separate cages and that never made physical contact.

#12 This is a new strain of Ebola, so what we know about other strains of Ebola may not necessarily apply to this strain of Ebola.

#13 Barack Obama has just signed an executive order that gives the federal government the power to apprehend and detain Americans that show symptoms of "diseases that are associated with fever and signs and symptoms of pneumonia or other respiratory illness, are capable of being transmitted from person to person, and that either are causing, or have the potential to cause, a pandemic, or, upon infection, are highly likely to cause mortality or serious morbidity if not properly controlled."

#14 And as I noted the other day, federal law already permits "the apprehension and examination of any individual reasonably believed to be infected with a communicable disease".

#15 According to the CDC, there are 20 quarantine centers around the country that are prepared to potentially receive Ebola patients...

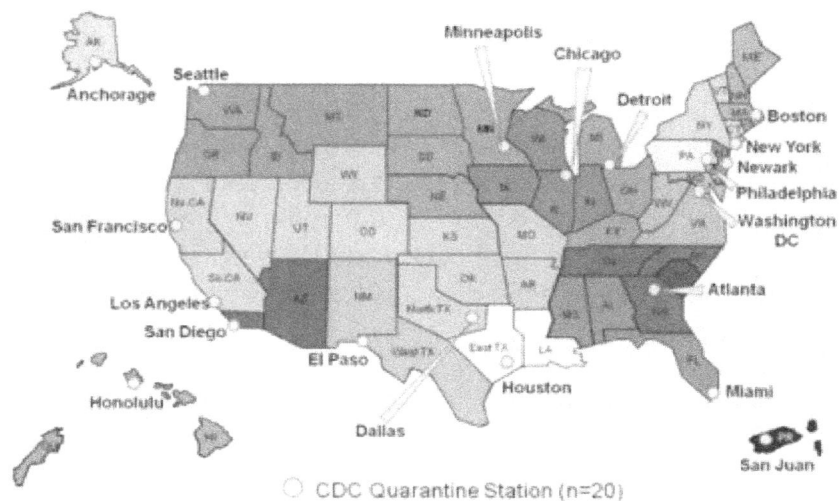

CDC Quarantine Station (n=20)

#16 The CDC has set up an Ebola "quarantine station" at LAX in order to help prevent the spread of the virus.

#17 The largest health emergency drill in New York City history was conducted on Friday.

#18 The federal government will begin testing an "experimental Ebola vaccine" on humans in September.

#19 We are being told that the reason why we don't have an Ebola vaccine already is due to the hesitation of the pharmaceutical industry to invest in a disease that has "only affected people in Africa".

#20 Researchers from Tulane University have been active for several years in the very same areas where this Ebola outbreak began. One of the stated purposes of this research was to study "the future use of fever-viruses as bioweapons".

#21 According to the Ministry of Health and Sanitation in Sierra Leone, researchers from Tulane University have been asked "to stop Ebola testing during the current Ebola outbreak". What in the world does that mean?

#22 The Navy Times says that the U.S. military has been interested in studying Ebola "as a potential biological weapon" since the 1970s...

Filoviruses like Ebola have been of interest to the Pentagon since the late 1970s, mainly because Ebola and its fellow viruses have high mortality rates — in the current outbreak, roughly 60 percent to 72 percent of those who have contracted the disease have died — and its stable nature in aerosol make it attractive as a potential biological weapon.

#23 The CDC actually owns a patent on one particular strain of the Ebola virus...

The U.S. Centers for Disease Control owns a patent on a particular strain of Ebola known as "EboBun." It's patent No. CA2741523A1 and it was awarded in 2010. You can view i t here.

It is being reported that this is not the same strain that is currently being transmitted in Africa, but it is interesting to note nonetheless. And why would the CDC want "ownership" of a strain of the Ebola virus in the first place?

#24 The CDC has just put up a brand new webpage entitled "Infection Prevention and Control Recommendations for Hospitalized Patients with Known or Suspected Ebola Hemorrhagic Fever in U.S. Hospitals".

#25 The World Health Organization has launched a 100 million dollar response plan to fight this Ebola outbreak. Others don't seem so alarmed. For example, Barack Obama is getting ready to take a "16 day Martha's Vineyard vacation".

Many are attempting to play down the threat from this virus by stating that unless you "exchange bodily fluids" with someone that you don't have anything to worry about.

If that was truly the case, then how in the world have more than 100 health workers contracted the virus so far?

Health professionals that deal with Ebola take extreme precautions to keep from being exposed to the disease.

But despite those extreme measures, they are catching it too.

So if this virus does start spreading all over the globe, what chance is the general population going to have?

Feel free to disagree with me if you like, but I believe that this could potentially be an absolutely catastrophic health crisis.

Hopefully I am wrong.

Michael Snyder

August 3rd, 2014

You can view this article at Michael's Website –

http://theeconomiccollapseblog.com/archives/25-critical-facts-about-this-ebola-outbreak-that-every-american-needs-to-know

APPENDIX B

Frequently asked questions on Ebola virus disease from WHO website

1. What is Ebola virus disease?

Ebola virus disease (formerly known as Ebola haemorrhagic fever) is a severe, often fatal illness, with a death rate of up to 90%. The illness affects humans and nonhuman primates (monkeys, gorillas, and chimpanzees).

Ebola first appeared in 1976 in two simultaneous outbreaks, one in a village near the Ebola River in the Democratic Republic of Congo, and the other in a remote area of Sudan.

The origin of the virus is unknown but fruit bats (Pteropodidae) are considered the likely host of the Ebola virus, based on available evidence.

2. How do people become infected with the virus?

Ebola is introduced into the human population through close contact with the blood, secretions, organs or other bodily fluids of infected animals. In Africa, infection has occurred through the handling of infected chimpanzees, gorillas, fruit bats, monkeys, forest antelope and porcupines found ill or dead or in the rainforest. It is important to reduce contact with high-risk animals (i.e. fruit bats, monkeys or apes) including not picking up dead animals found lying in the forest or handling their raw meat.

Once a person comes into contact with an animal that has Ebola, it can spread within the community from human to human. Infection occurs from direct contact (through broken skin or mucous membranes) with the blood, or other bodily fluids or secretions (stool, urine, saliva, semen) of infected people. Infection can also occur if broken skin or mucous membranes of a healthy person come into contact with environments that have become contaminated with an Ebola patient's infectious fluids such as soiled clothing, bed linen, or used needles.

Health workers have frequently been exposed to the virus when caring for Ebola patients. This happens because they are not wearing personal protection equipment, such as gloves, when caring for the patients. Health care providers at all levels of the health system – hospitals, clinics and health posts – should be briefed on the nature of the disease and how it is transmitted, and strictly follow recommended infection control precautions.

Burial ceremonies in which mourners have direct contact with the body of the deceased person can also play a role in the transmission of Ebola. Persons who have died of Ebola must be handled using strong protective clothing and gloves, and be buried immediately.

People are infectious as long as their blood and secretions contain the virus. For this reason, infected patients receive close monitoring from medical professionals and receive laboratory tests to ensure the virus is no longer circulating in their systems before they return home. When the medical professionals determine it is okay for the patient to return home, they are no longer infectious and cannot infect anyone else in their communities. Men who have recovered from the illness can still spread the virus to their partner through their semen for up to 7 weeks after recovery. For this reason, it is important for men to avoid sexual intercourse for at least 7 weeks after recovery or to wear condoms if having sexual intercourse during 7 weeks after recovery.

3. Who is most at risk?

During an outbreak, those at higher risk of infection are:

health workers;

family members or others in close contact with infected people;

mourners who have direct contact with the bodies of the deceased as part of burial ceremonies; and hunters in the rain forest who come into contact with dead animals found lying in the forest.

More research is needed to understand if some groups, such as immuno-compromised people or those with other underlying health conditions, are more susceptible than others to contracting the virus.

Exposure to the virus can be controlled through the use of protective measures in clinics and hospitals, at community gatherings, or at home.

4. What are typical signs and symptoms of infection?

Sudden onset of fever, intense weakness, muscle pain, headache and sore throat are typical signs and symptoms. This is followed by vomiting, diarrhoea, rash, impaired kidney and liver function, and in some cases, both internal and external bleeding.

Laboratory findings include low white blood cell and platelet counts, and elevated liver enzymes.

The incubation period, or the time interval from infection to onset of symptoms, is from 2 to 21 days. The patients become contagious once they begin to show symptoms. They are not contagious during the incubation period.

Ebola virus disease infections can only be confirmed through laboratory testing.

5. When should someone seek medical care?

If a person has been in an area known to have Ebola virus disease or in contact with a person known or suspected to have Ebola and they begin to have symptoms, they should seek medical care immediately.

Any cases of persons who are suspected to have the disease should be reported to the nearest health unit without delay. Prompt medical care is essential to improving the rate of survival from the disease. It is also important to control spread of the disease and infection control procedures need to be started immediately.

6. What is the treatment?

Severely ill patients require intensive supportive care. They are frequently dehydrated and need intravenous fluids or oral rehydration with solutions that contain electrolytes. There is currently no specific treatment to cure the disease.

Some patients will recover with the appropriate medical care.

To help control further spread of the virus, people that are suspected or confirmed to have the disease should be isolated from other patients and treated by health workers using strict infection control precautions.

7. What can I do? Can Ebola be prevented?

Currently there is no licensed vaccine for Ebola virus disease. Several vaccines are being tested, but none are available for clinical use right now.

Raising awareness of the risk factors and measures people can take to protect themselves are the only ways to reduce illness and deaths.

Ways to prevent infection and transmission

While initial cases of Ebola virus disease are contracted by handling infected animals or carcasses, secondary cases occur by direct contact with the bodily fluids of an ill person, either through unsafe case management or unsafe burial practices. *During this outbreak, most of the disease has spread through human-to-human transmission*. Several steps can be taken to help in preventing infection and limiting or stopping transmission.

Understand the nature of the disease, how it is transmitted, and how to prevent it from spreading further. (For additional information, please see the previous questions about Ebola virus disease in this FAQ.)

Listen to and follow directives issued by your country's respective Ministry of Health.

If you suspect someone close to you or in your community of having Ebola virus disease, encourage and support them in seeking appropriate medical treatment in a care facility.

If you choose to care for an ill person in your home, notify public health officials of your intentions so they can train you and provide appropriate gloves and personal protective equipment (PPE), as well as instructions as a reminder on how to properly care for the patient, protect yourself and your family, and properly dispose of the PPE after use.

When visiting patients in the hospital or caring for someone at home, hand washing with soap and water is recommended after touching a patient, being in contact with their bodily fluids, or touching his/her surroundings.

People who have died from Ebola should only be handled using appropriate protective equipment and should be buried immediately.

Additionally, individuals should reduce contact with high-risk infected animals (i.e. fruit bats, monkeys or apes) in the affected rainforest areas. If you suspect an animal is infected, do not handle it. Animal products (blood and meat) should be thoroughly cooked before eating.

8. What about health workers? How do they protect themselves from the high risk of caring for sick patients?

Health workers treating patients with suspected or confirmed illness are at higher risk of infection than other groups.

In addition to standard health care precautions, health workers should strictly apply recommended infection control measures to avoid exposure to infected blood, fluids, or contaminated environments or objects – such as a patient's soiled linen or used needles.

They should use personal protection equipment such as individual gowns, gloves, masks and goggles or face shields.

They should not reuse protective equipment or clothing unless they have been properly disinfected.

They should change gloves between caring for each patient suspected of having Ebola.

Invasive procedures that can expose medical doctors, nurses and others to infection should be carried out under strict, safe conditions.

Infected patients should be kept separate from other patients and healthy people, as much as possible.

9. What about rumours that some foods can prevent or treat the infection?

WHO strongly recommends that people seek credible health advice about Ebola virus disease from their public health authority.

While there is no specific drug against Ebola, the best treatment is intensive supportive treatment provided in the hospital by health workers using strict infection control procedures. The infection can be controlled through recommended protective measures.

10. How does WHO protect health during outbreaks?

WHO provides technical advice to countries and communities to prepare for and respond to Ebola outbreaks.

WHO actions include:

- disease surveillance and information-sharing across regions to watch for outbreaks;

- technical assistance to investigate and contain health threats when they occur – such as on-site help to identify sick people and track disease patterns;
- advice on prevention and treatment options;
- deployments of experts and the distribution of health supplies (such as personal protection gear for health workers) when they are requested by the country;
- communications to raise awareness of the nature of the disease and protective health measures to control transmission of the virus; and
- activation of regional and global networks of experts to provide assistance, if requested, and mitigate potential international health effects and disruptions of travel and trade.

11. During an outbreak, numbers of cases reported by health officials can go up and down? Why?

During an Ebola outbreak, the affected country's public health authority reports its disease case numbers and deaths. Figures can change daily. Case numbers reflect both suspected cases and laboratory-confirmed cases of Ebola. Sometimes numbers of suspected and confirmed cases are reported together. Sometimes they are reported separately. Thus, numbers can shift between suspected and confirmed cases.

Analyzing case data trends, over time, and with additional information, is generally more helpful to assess the public health situation and determine the appropriate response.

12. Is it safe to travel during an outbreak? What is WHO's travel advice?

During an outbreak, WHO reviews the public health situation regularly, and recommends any travel or trade restrictions if necessary.

The risk of infection for travelers is very low since person-to-person transmission results from direct contact with the body fluids or secretions of an infected patient.

WHO's general travel advice

Travelers should avoid all contact with infected patients.

Health workers traveling to affected areas should strictly follow WHO-recommended infection control guidance.

Anyone who has stayed in areas where cases were recently reported should be aware of the symptoms of infection and seek medical attention at the first sign of illness.

Clinicians caring for travelers returning from affected areas with compatible symptoms are advised to consider the possibility of Ebola virus disease.

Endnotes:

(1) http://www.acponline.org/pressroom/pan_flu.htm

(2) http://afludiary.blogspot.com/2008/03/ventilator-triage-during-pandemic.html

(1) http://charlotte.cbslocal.com/2014/07/31/liberian-official-ebola-outbreak-is-above-the-control-of-the-national-government/

(2) http://www.phac-aspc.gc.ca/lab-bio/res/psds-ftss/ebola-eng.php

(3) http://www.kefir.net/what-is-kefir/

(4) https://suite.io/sara-mcgrath/64vf290

(5) http://www.mayoclinic.org/diseases-conditions/dehydration/basics/symptoms/con-20030056

(6) http://www.who.int/water_sanitation_health/hygiene/envsan/tn08/en/

=-=-=-=-=-=-=-=-=-=-=-=

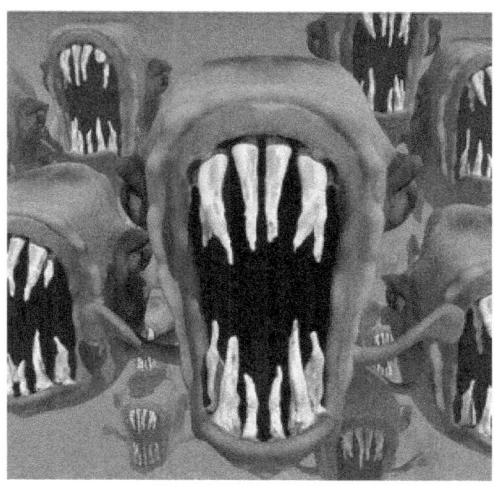

Ebola Virus Gone Wild

CPSIA information can be obtained
at www.ICGtesting.com
Printed in the USA
LVHW081624270220
648396LV00016B/783

9 781502 844903